STEPS FOR DISEASE PREVENTION AND HEALTHY LIVING

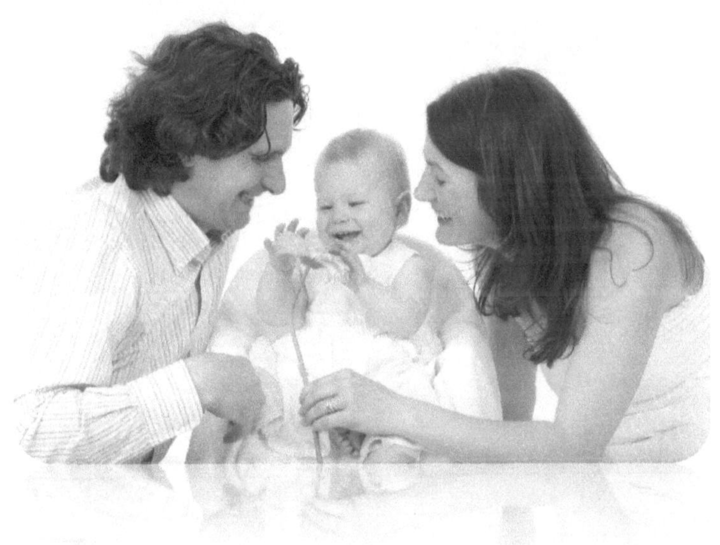

Content

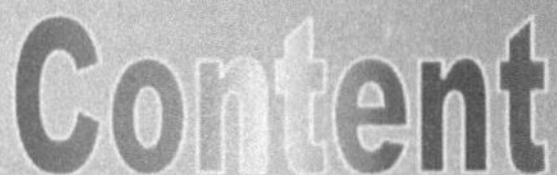

Introduction

Care of the psychological state

Tips for Health Care

Practesing Sports

Slimming and fitness

INTRODUCTION

Health is one of the important things for every living organism is the basis of the global system, a healthy person well-being can do all his duty and his responsibility and follow his life with ease unlike a sick person or who is not in good health is unable to do any work and be frozen is not useful in any One thing is that care for health is a duty of every person and a direct responsibility of families to protect their children and keep them safe. To help you with this, you can use and dependence this companion "Steps for Disease Prevention and Healthy Living" to help you on this task and show you the best ways to prevent .

The responsibility of the individual to take care of health Begins from birth, and the mother and family take care of it at that stage When a person begins to grow and know everything around him, he begins to be cautious in his steps and soon realizes the dangers of some things , When a person reaches puberty, he is mature enough to take care of himself and know the importance of maintaining health and preventing diseases and other things that pose a threat to the safety of himself and unable to produce and follow his life as a result of the deterioration of his health .

In this case, the person begins the best ways and ways to prevent diseases and maintain health, it is a good initiative of everyone and in our interesting and concise book we will talk about the factors that make you healthy and well-being and enable you to follow your life well .

WHY I SHOULD BE TAKE CARE OF MY HEALTH?

Health means being able to follow up on your work and face problems and the ability to solve them as well as to help you follow your life without stress , You should also be in good health to carry out the duties that you and the care of your family and ensure its responsibility and maintain health in simple ways uncomplicated and comfortable, the simplest ways can be followed and in this book we will show you the best ways to maintain physical health and mental health and get rid of stressors, all in a fun and easy way .

BENEFITS OF MAINTAINING HEALTH:

After learning about the importance of maintaining health I will give you several benefits and reasons to be more interested in maintaining your health and take it seriously and give it more importance.

SUCCESS IN YOUR WORK FIELD:

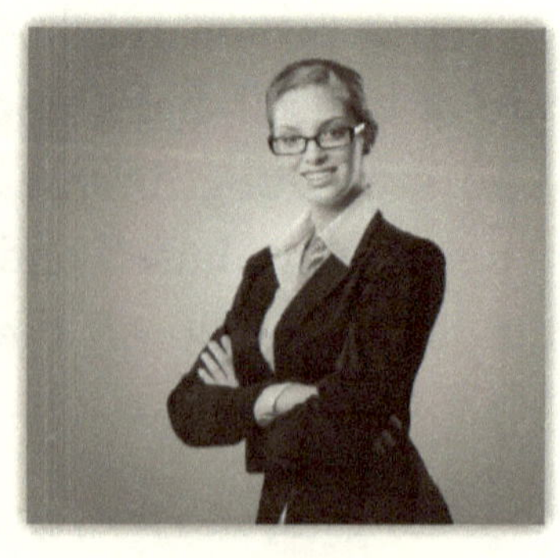

A healthy mind in a healthy body and good health means efficiency in the performance of business, if you maintain your health and take care of yourself you will be able to accomplish your work and follow-up and thus be successful and independent in your work , and become a dependable employee in the company, and you may get rewards and more for the efforts they provide and the basis in that being Because you has a healthy person , It also makes you loved by company members and employer , but If your health is in a bad situation, you will not be able to continue your job or accomplish any work, but you may lose your job as a result of failing to do your work, so it is better to start now to follow the best ways to protect and protect yourself .

CARE FOR YOUR FAMILY:

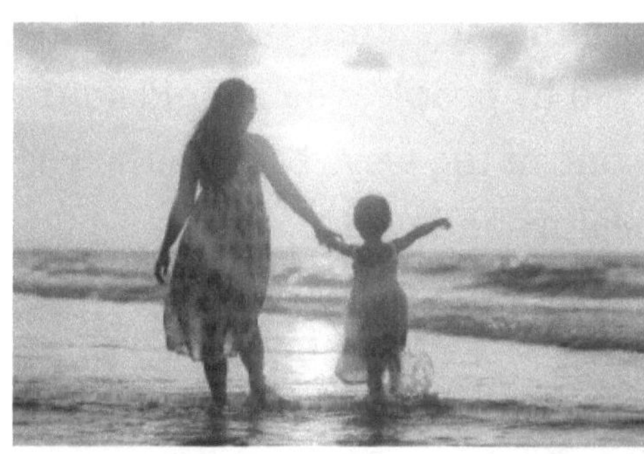

Have you ever thought about what will happen to your family members without being near them and support them, of course, their situation will be very bad and unimaginable and to care for your family you must be healthy and well-being so you can provide them with all the support they need and therefore care for health is a duty , also You are considered a lunch for your family members and therefore should be an example of self-care , It is also your direct responsibility to protect the health of your children, so you should know how to protect them from disease , and You should be aware of ways to care for children and young people and to do so you must be healthy in the first place .

MAKE YOU LOVELY AMONG PEOPLE:

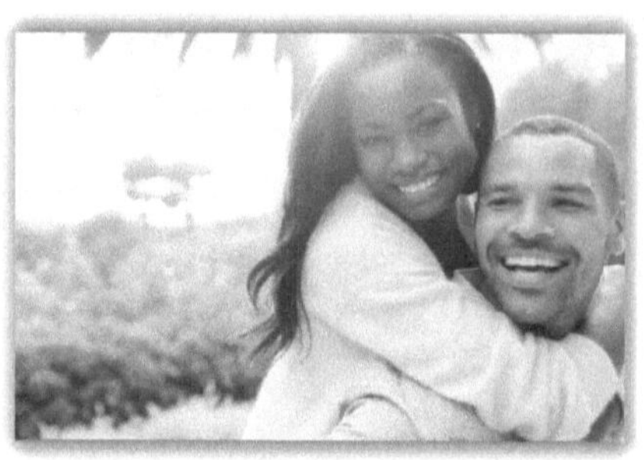

A healthy person will always be loved by people and find everyone approaching him and trying to form a relationship with him, Reverse person whose health is deteriorating or in poor condition, there is no interest from people. People consider a healthy person as a source of inspiration for them as well as being reliable in performing any kind of work , So if you're looking for ways to be loved by people, you should start to keep you healthy, Because It is one of the ways besides the good appearance that you will look healthy and well .

MAKE OFFER WONDERFUL TO YOUR LIFE PARTNER:

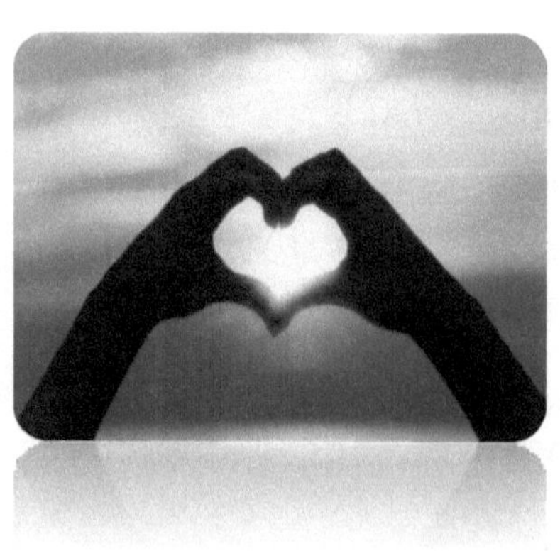

Do you know what is the closest thing to your partner and makes it related to you in larger images, certainly it is Intimate relationship is one of the most things that increase the bond between the two partners and strengthen their relationship , The opposite can be said that the inability to keep up with a life partner during Intimate relationship and ED causes a weak relationship between the two partners and makes you in an awkward position , and To be able to provide convincing performance in bed, you must be a healthy and healthy person who determines your effectiveness during intimacy, and for this reason you must take care of your health .

EXCELLENCE IN STUDY:

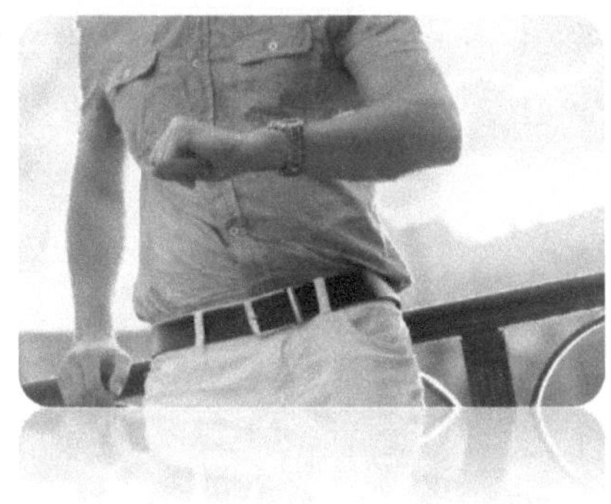

If you are a student in different stages of education, you should look for the best ways to excel in your studies and ensure a brilliant future full of interaction, and good health is one of the key factors that ensure you success in your educational attainment and achieve good results, if you are healthy, it means you are able to Focus on your lessons , by this way, you can outperform your classmates and be able to achieve amazing results, but for a person who lacks good health cannot expect from him positive results and return all this backfired undesirable because he could not focus on his lessons because of the deterioration of his condition .

MAINTAINING HEALTH MAKES YOU AN ATTRACTIVE GUY:

If you are young at the beginning of your life, maintaining health is one of the important and necessary things that you should pay attention to, your health means your attractiveness, so you should always try to show the best condition in addition to take care of your physical health is one of the main features of the young man , also, if you have a good fitness and a strong body makes you attractive for girls and quickly gather around you and get close to you, and this is loved by every young man so my advice to you, young man, your health means your personality and your eyes, which is what matters to people so you have to pay attention to your physical health .

MAINTAINING HEALTH MAKES YOU AN ATTRACTIVE GIRL:

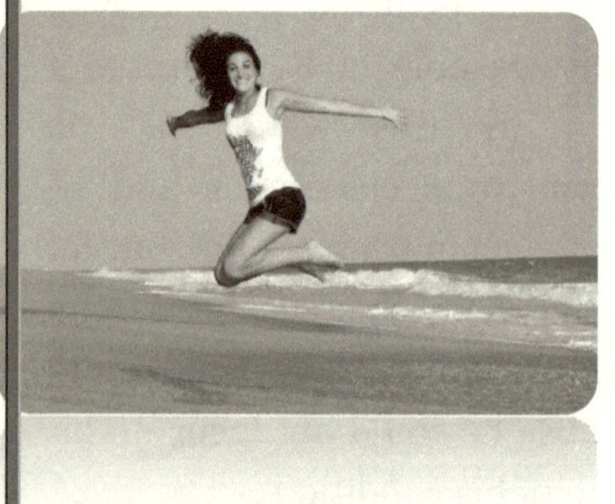

As such maintaining health is important for guy and make it more attractive, it also includes you, taking care of health is important for every young girl who wants to enjoy her life, it is your priorities to maintain the health of your body and fitness , As well as taking care of your beauty and taking care of your personality and these things make you attractive and capturing the eyes of any guy easily, and other features of health care is to make you loved among your friends and boast of them and enjoy the spirit of fun and passion and thus impress anyone.

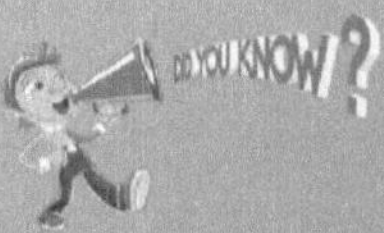

DO YOU KNOW

- Did you know that breast milk contains immunity protect the child and maintain his health without the need for other preventive methods

- Did you know that the number of heart valves in the human body four and the number of normal heartbeats 72 pulse

- Did you know that a person can mute or lock himself for 3 to 7 minutes

HEALTH AND FAMILY

IF YOU ARE A RESPONSIBLE PERSON AND YOU HAVE A FAMILY UNDER YOUR RESPONSIBILITY THEN YOU NEED TO KNOW ALL THE DIFFERENT HEALTH AND PREVENTIVE METHODS, THEN YOU ARE A RESPONSIBLE OF PROTECTING YOUR FAMILY AND KEEPING THEM SAFE FROM HEALTH RISKS AND VARIOUS DISEASES , AND TO ACHIEVE THIS YOU HAVE TO BE LOOKING AT ABOUT ALL THE HEALTH CARE AND KEEP A REGULAR FOLLOW-UP OF DOCTORS AND CONSULT THEM TO SHOW YOU THAT THE BEST THINGS THAT HELP TO PROTECT YOUR FAMILY AND KEEP THEM SAFE , AND HERE ARE SOME GUIDELINES THAT WILL HELP YOU DO THIS FIRST , AS WELL AS TAKING CARE OF YOUR CHILDREN AND CONDUCTING TESTS FOR THEM ON AN ONGOING BASIS , KEEPING THE HOUSE CLEAN AND DISINFECTING HELPS REDUCE DISEASES AND KILL BACTERIA , AS WELL AS ATTENTION TO PERSONAL HYGIENE OF CHILDREN AND FAMILY MEMBERS, WHICH MAKES THEM MORE IMMUNE AGAINST VARIOUS DISEASES .

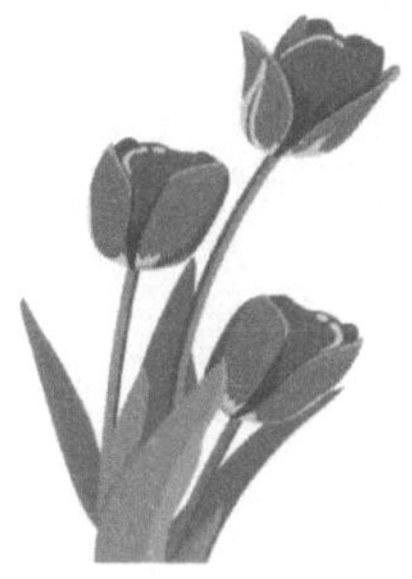
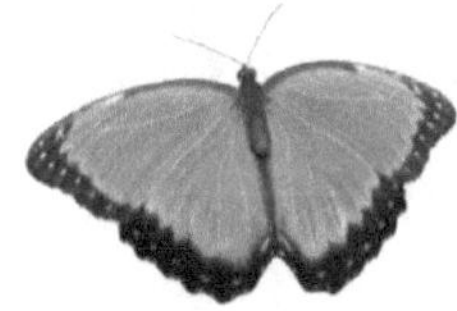
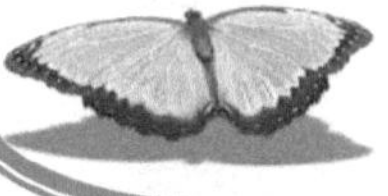

Man without hope as a plant without water and man without a smile as a rose without smell , Experience is the comb that life gives you when you have lost your hair , You may endure pain for hours, but do not accept to be desperate even for a moment , And ambition is what helps man to reach success, and there is no elevator for success, but there is a ladder you climb

TIPS FOR PSYCHOLOGICAL HEALTH

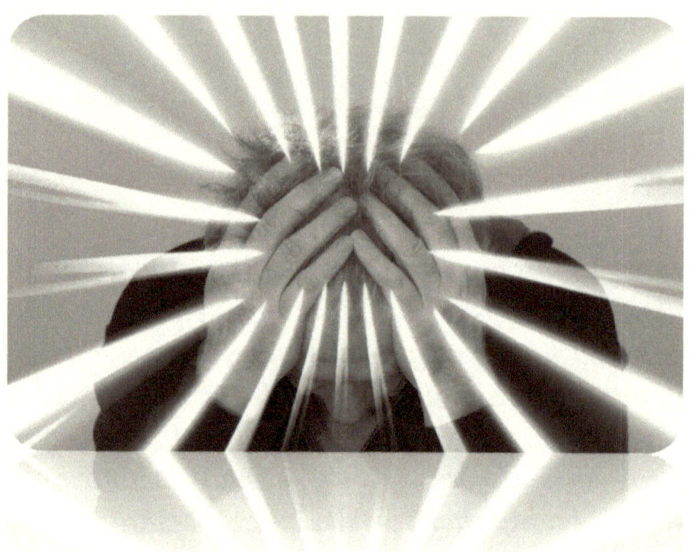

The psychological state or mood is one of the most important things that affect the abilities of any person was so in order to achieve full care for the health of ourselves must start from the psychological state , Mood Effect a direct way to our behavior and different behaviors and way of living our lives, a person with a moderate mood find a center and follower of his work and his life, while the person who suffers from the strikes and psychological pressures you find hardly feel things around him and find it always late that the rest of the people , Therefore, we should not underestimate the psychological state and mood and its impact on us, so any individual should pay attention to his mood and modify it and try to get rid of the pressures of different life and face it with all sensibility , The main idea to take care of the mood is to relax and not to think deeply that will overburden the mind and make it start with a backlash as a result of excessive thinking .

As for the problems of life, who does not mean them, there is almost no person in this world who does not have problems in his life, but this does not mean that we integrate into these problems and tire ourselves in dealing with them, but it is sufficient for us to gradually solve them without harming ourselves and our mental health, so there is always a side Bright and dark in life, and this does not mean that we always choose the difficult way to solve things. It is sufficient for us to deal with those problems slowly and spontaneously and choose the most appropriate way that does not harm us .

Among the other things that are considered one of the main problems facing some people are the expectations that people and members of your family expect from you, so we notice that this person seemed to pressure himself to achieve those expectations that were set for him and he is not the one who chose it for himself and this is not a healthy way at all .

And now, after learning about the importance of mental health care, I will provide you with a set of tips and instructions that will help you greatly in maintaining your mental health and getting rid of the pressures that are inherent to you. You only need to apply these instructions and you will notice a big difference in your life.

DON'T DEEPER INTO THINKING:

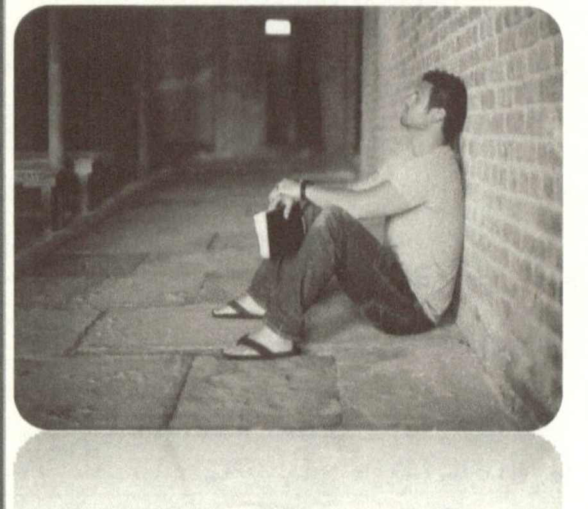

Did you know that most people with mental illness were thinking was the first reason for bringing this disease or was a primary reason for that, in addition to that most people who think deeply suffer from bad mood and malaise , In addition to many problems and diseases that bring you in-depth thinking, it is here that you reduce the occupancy rate of your mind and give it periods of rest, in addition to the pressures and problems of life and enjoy flexibility in facing problems of various kinds, and give the mind a little pleasure and fun that it deserves by enjoying your life and giving yourself a chance to vent As for her income .

HOPE AND OPTIMISM:

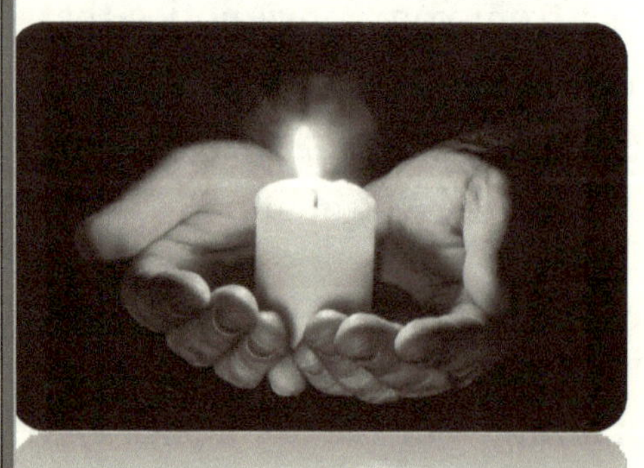

One of the great secrets that people hear constantly, but consider it just words it is the hope, do you know that a person can endure days and hours of hunger, thirst, disease and perhaps pain, but he cannot bear the simplest things, which is the loss of hope and disappointment, even for a moment , Because hope has a direct relationship to the health condition and the psychological state in the first place, and the same thing can be said that optimism and therefore your view of life must be a positive view and try to sense the white side of life, and not to think and see things always with a negative view which leads to harm your mental health .

VISIT A PSYCHOLOGY DOCTOR:

It is not necessary for you to be a psychopath to visit a psychiatrist, as this behavior is normal and good for you , Visiting the psychiatrist gives you a lot of benefits in addition to the valuable directions that you will get from the specialized doctor and it is also an opportunity to breathe that self, so visit the psychiatrist frequently from period to time, and encourage yourself to confront doctors and integrate with them, and soon you will find a clear improvement in your psychological condition .

SPENDING TIME WITH FRIENDS:

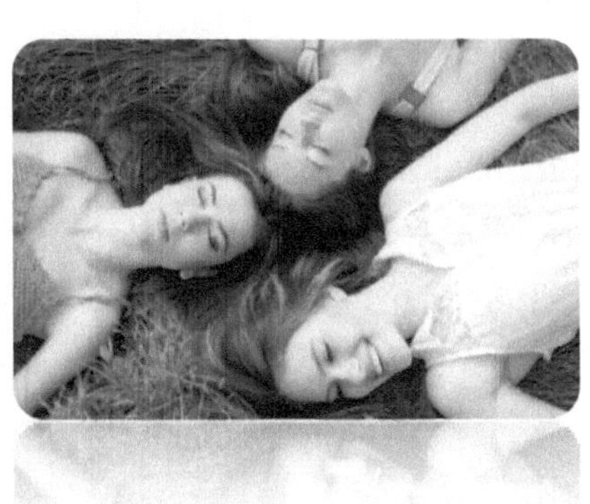

It is also considered one of the best ways to maintain mental health and modify moods and behaviors, so you should devote some time to sitting and chatting with your friends or family members and sharing all your problems with them and this will work to gradually improve your mood and maintain your mental health .

LISTENING TO MUSIC:

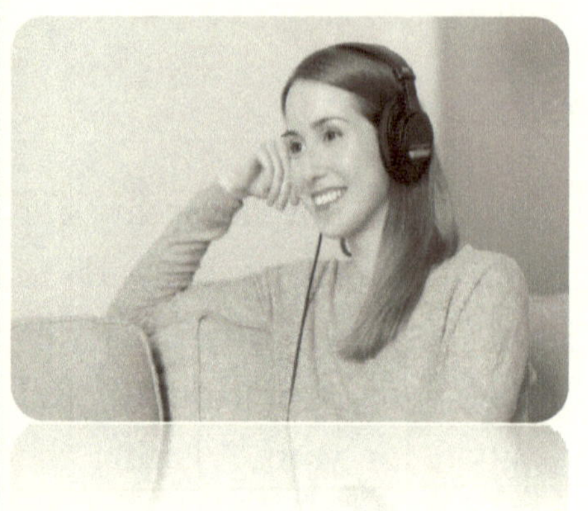

Do you realize that music has a special effect on the psyche of any person and a profound impact within it, as music is one of the therapeutic methods for cases of misery and depression , And it is approved by doctors in improving the psychological state, so you should relax and listen to music. It is not meant for loud music but rather quiet music that interferes with pleasure in the heart, so we advise you to listen to music from time to time and enjoy it.

MEDITATION:

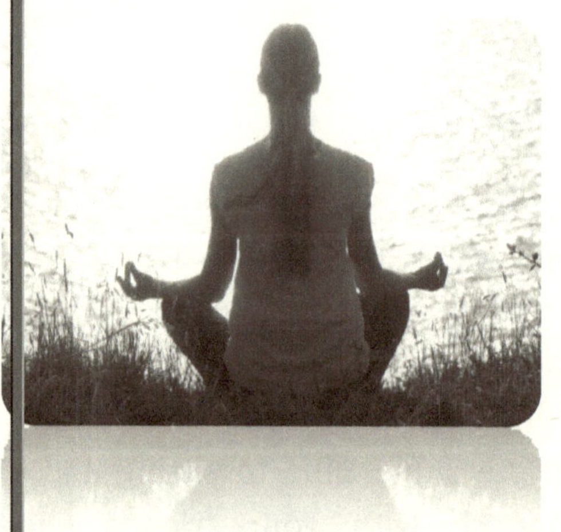

Meditation is considered one of the best ways to prevent mental illnesses, and that, in the case of work, there is a connection between him and his inner self, and as a result he exits all the negative energy and is filled with interaction and vitality , and To protect your health and protect the psychological state, you must set aside time and sit between you and yourself, contemplate the scenes or anything that leads to interaction .

DO NOT BE HOSTILE:

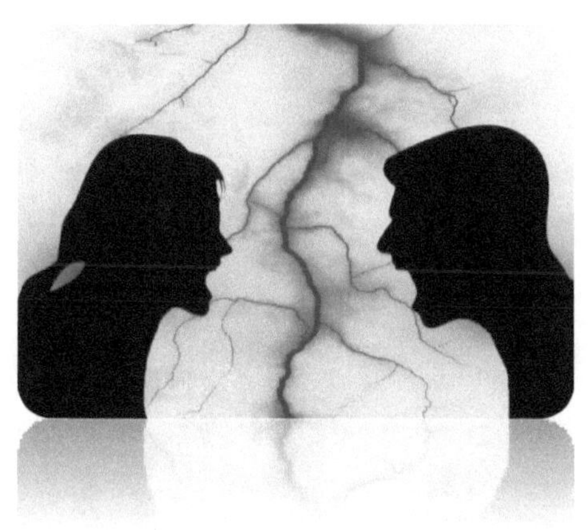

The hostile personality poses a risk to the mental health of any person and leads to psychological strikes and hallucinations, and to protect your mental health you have to be a spontaneous person and better behave with people and thus become loved by them.

In addition, the aggressive person cannot perform any kind of business or achieve success in his life, and you find him constantly complaining and angry at the simplest things and this is not a completely healthy way.

TIPS FOR HEALTH CARE

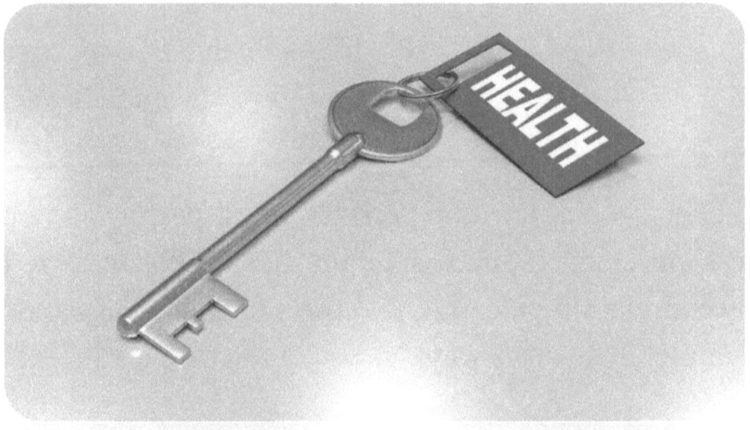

We have reached a new stage in our interesting book and have learned the benefits of maintaining health and have identified the most important things that help you maintain health , In this chapter, I have devoted a wide range of tips and methods that will help you to preserve your health and live in peace of mind , In addition, these instructions are recognized by doctors and are considered a valuable treasure for the sake of maintaining health. Have you heard the saying that "prevention is better than cure" This proverb has very many meanings and a more meaningful meaning that can be interpreted. Do not wait for the disease until it affects you and then start With treatment, the right thing is to protect and protect yourself from disease even before it hits you, and this is the right healthy way.

Now without delay, I will put in place tips and plans to preserve your health and the health of your family and guarantee you complete prevention and safety from diseases. All you have to do is to apply these instructions and soon you will notice a big difference in your life, so let's get lost .

GOOD DIET:

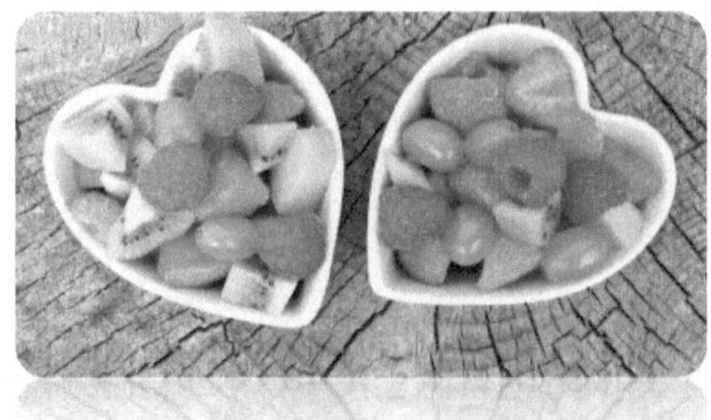

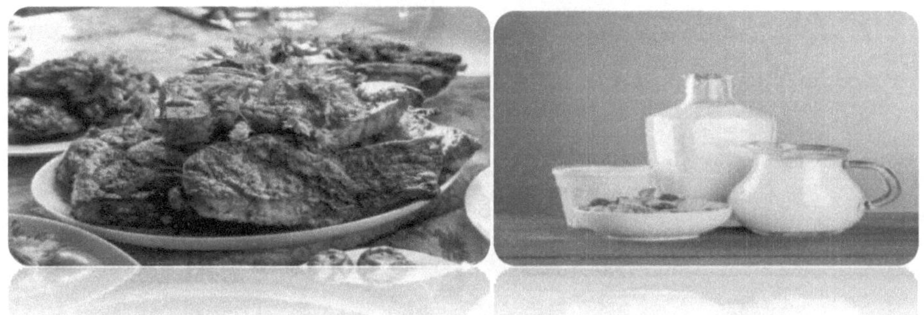

Nutrition is the basis of life for all living organisms and is considered the most important thing for a person. Food would provide the body with energy and help it to carry out its tasks and move forward in his life, and it is impossible for any person to dispense with food as it is the basic factor of life and without it a person cannot live, Of course, food varies greatly in terms of its shape, taste, and type, and each variety has its own advantages and benefits that you do not find at another type of food, in addition to the fact that human health is directly affected by the type of food and diet that a person follows, so you have to choose good foods that will benefit your body and health And I do not mean that you adhere to a certain type of food or follow any diet, so love is food grown for every person, regardless of his personality, you can eat everything that you like, but in balanced amounts, so that this behavior will not return you negative results on your health .

One of the important foods that you must make sure to eat constantly is the fresh fruits, as it contains many vitamins and glucose that supply the body with energy, and it cannot be denied that eating meat helps in building the body and its cohesion, and among the important foods is milk and is considered one of the most important types of food as it provides the body with the energy it needs Other than his other benefits, such as building bones, therefore it is advised to drink milk daily, especially for children, to help them grow and increase their immunity against diseases .

TRY A BANANA MILK RECIPE

A very useful recipe for human health and helps in the growth of the body and the preservation of health. It can also be presented to children who do not like to drink milk. It is delicious and thus helps them to benefit from the benefits found in milk as well as the description , The method of preparation is very easy, two cups of milk and one banana you mix and filter and have your meal ready .

Some people think that sweets and pastries are harmful to health, but there are no harmful foods unless a person overindulges them and therefore it is advised to eat pastries and sweets in small quantities because they contain the sugar that the body needs but it is not necessary to overeat them, in addition because there are many foods that we cannot limit all of them What is important is that we know that food has an important role in maintaining health and therefore every person must follow a good and varied diet .

As for stimulants such as tea, coffee, etc., it is okay to drink them, as there are many benefits that the body benefits from, such as caffeine, but it is not recommended that a person get used to drinking them in large quantities, this leads to harm to health, so if you are used to drinking these stimuli, you should be careful and reduce them and it is not advised to give them For children and young people.

CARRYING OUT MEDICAL EXAMINATIONS:

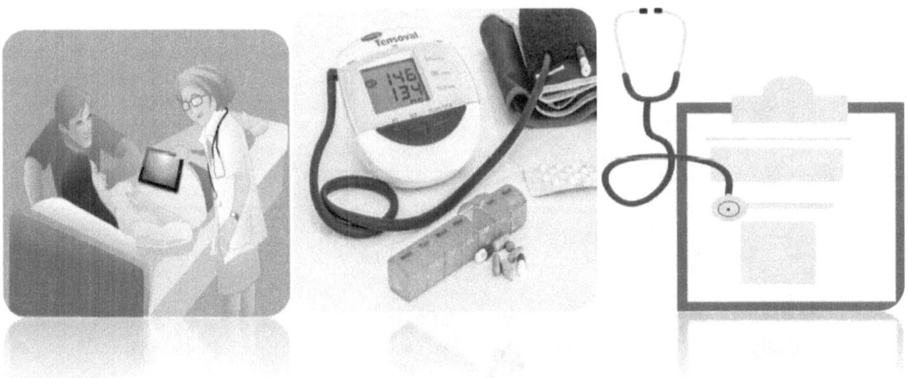

Conducting medical examinations is a normal and routine matter. It is very important to do these exams. It shows you all the problems that determine your health and well-being and gives you a way to prevent diseases before you get sick. It is also important for medical exams to give you complete information that the health condition is yours , So you are aware of the level of blood pressure and the level of sugar in the blood is it high or low and what are the vitamins that your body needs in addition to other benefits, so you have to do Medical examinations for you and your family, this helps a lot in maintaining health and safety from diseases .

And do not forget to set a schedule for visiting the doctor, for example, once a week, once a month, and so on, so that you do not forget about it.

QUIT THE BAD HABITS:

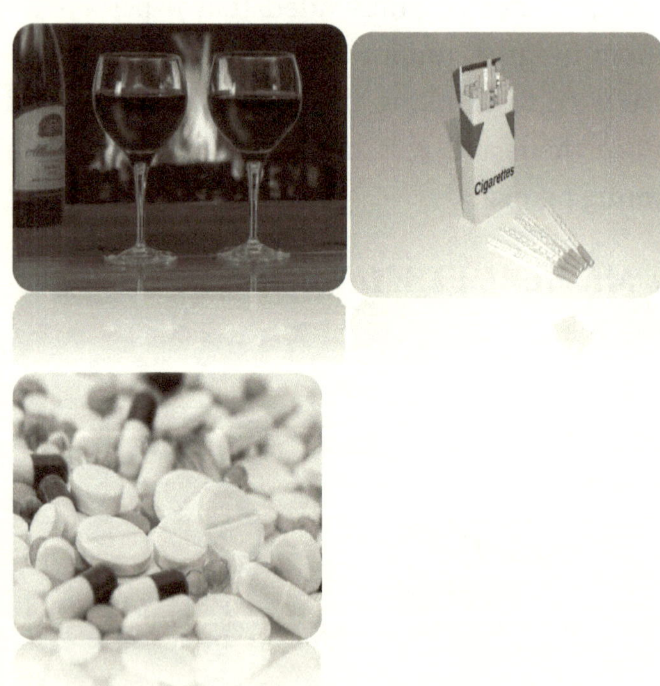

Quitting or leaving bad and harmful habits is considered the most important advice that I want to offer you dear reader, there are a lot of things harmful to health as a result of these harmful practices , and the first of these habits is smoking, which has become widely spread among people, and there are many reasons that make anyone have a good reason to leave this practice in addition to the great health risks of this behavior. We must not forget the serious diseases that smoking brings, including cancer , Therefore, you should quit smoking, even if gradually, as this would protect your health and safety , And one of the practices that must be abandoned is also the drinking of alcohol and intoxicants, which is also common. These intoxicants have many harmful effects on health and cause gradually weakening and demolishing the body and soon the person becomes vulnerable to the spreading diseases, in addition to the fact that alcohol exceeds the harm to physical health and causes great harm to mental health and causes strikes, hallucinations and other harm Mental , , So from my point of view it should be left completely healthy Living is better than getting fun hours and spend the rest of your life infected with diseases .

As for children, it is preferable that there be control by them from parents, this would protect your family members from diseases, as well as there are many wrong practices that you should beware of and leave them in case you feel that they are harmful to your general health .

DRINKING WATER:

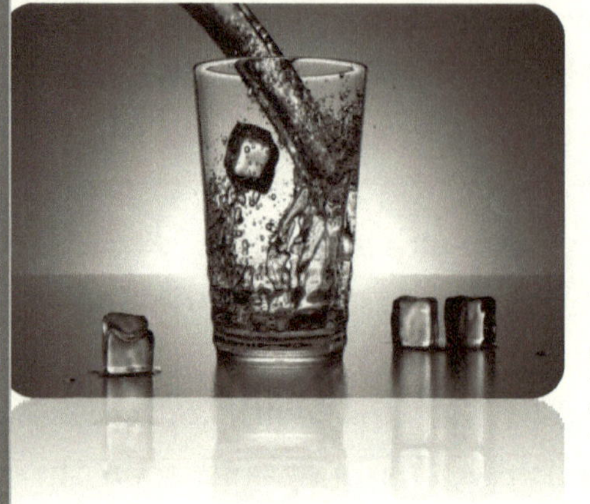

Drinking water has benefits for maintaining health in its own right. Water is the basic factor upon which the global system is based. No living creature can dispense or live without water, Water also has many benefits, and so it represents a large part of the human formation and is considered more important than food. Even in order to maintain healthy health, it is necessary to drink large quantities of water every day as it helps the person to digest and distribute food inside the body and makes the person more vital, You can also benefit from water in other ways, such as taking a warm bath or steam bath, as well as swimming, to help maintain vitality and vitality.

WATCH MOVIES:

I still remember that scene from the movie "Central Intelligence" starring Doyon Jason "The Rock" and Kevin Hart. The scene was that Kevin Hart's wife, the role of Calvin Junior, suggested that he visit the psychiatrist after the relationship between them deteriorated, so he told her we Samar do not visit psychiatrists Rather, we go to the barber shop to talk about our problems or watch a movie , This section of the movie made me laugh for a few minutes, so from my point of view watching the films is good and delighting in the soul, in addition to the valuable benefits that we gain from them, Also, there are a lot of cinematic works that send pleasure in the soul and take you to the world of imagination and fun in the soul and forget the concerns of life and encourage you to move forward, Also this reminded me of " The greatest show man " starring Hugh Jack man and the movie is very beautiful and it tells about the difficulties and problems of life and how the person encounters it so I advise you to watch it , The bottom line is that watching movies is a kind of catharsis that is self and beneficial to health, so you can relax and watch movies from time to time.

GOOD SLEEP:

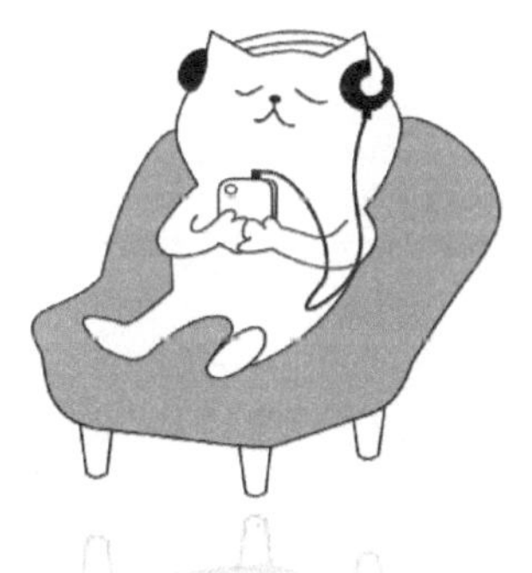

An important advice to maintain health and enjoy a strong and resilient body is good deep sleep, as it helps to relax the internal organs of the human being and makes them renew their activities in addition to maintaining mental and psychological health , Because a person who does not sleep well finds him exhausted most of the time and cannot perform his work in an acceptable manner unlike the person who sleeps well so you find him active and performs his duty to the fullest, therefore my advice to you is good sleep and not magic or work until late hours of the night, this would harm Your health, so divide your time and save part of your personal comfort.

And from the quick advice that I want to offer you, I get some fun and enjoyment, because it is one of the things that enters pleasure in the soul and makes you less vulnerable to the spreading diseases such as the caliphate and others, So I make sure to go out what your friends and fun and joke with them and thus be healthy and exempt, and you can also invent ways that you think are appropriate to preserve your health.

PRACTICING SPORTS

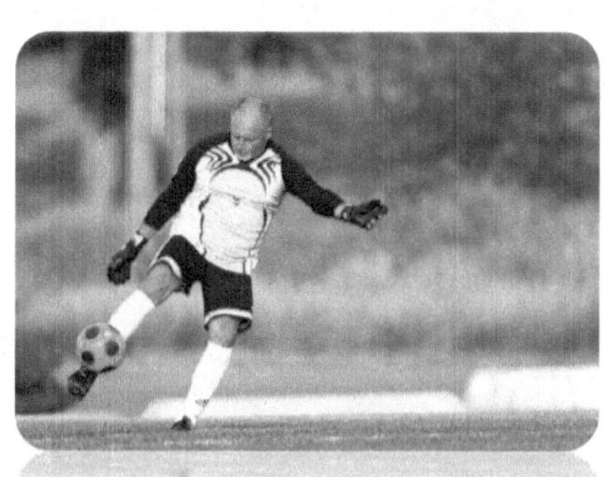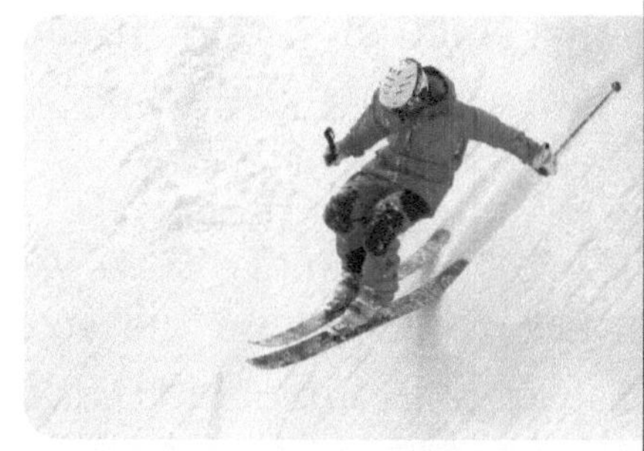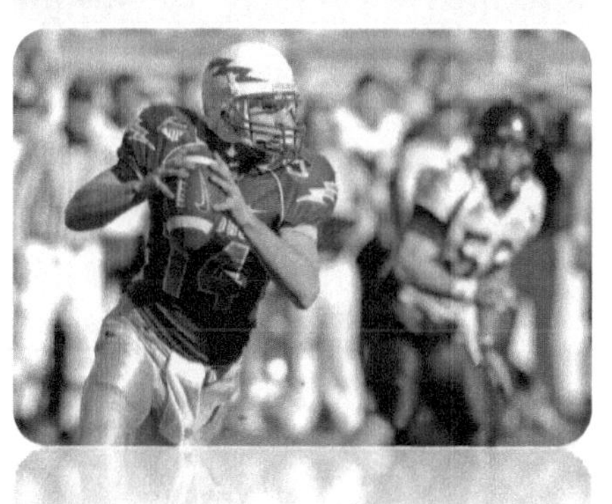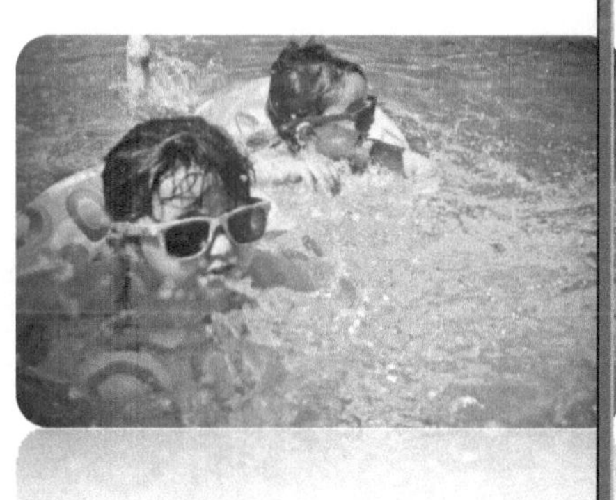

Sport has a direct relationship to human health and safety besides the valuable benefits, as sport represents the backbone on which the rest of the body is concentrated, so sport is important for any male or female, large or small because sport represents a large role in maintaining health and keeping the body straight from disease in addition to side benefits Such as improving body fitness and getting fit and attractive appearance , Therefore, in this chapter we will show the best sports that you can practice that will help you in maintaining your health and staying safe from diseases, as well as showing the types of sports that children can practice and are safe for them and useful , But first, let's get to know the benefits of exercising quickly:

>> Maintaining the health and general activity of the body as it renews the activity of the body and increases the speed of its interaction with movement.

>> Getting fit and perfect body This is the best thing you may need after maintaining your health and safety.

>> Having fun and reducing stress, so it is a good idea to exercise after every hard day of work until you get active again.

>> It helps you focus as it activates all the cells of the body, including the cells of the mind, which is the center of thinking and focus.

>> Also, sport helps a person to sleep deeply and it is what helps a person to maintain his health as we mentioned earlier.

>> It makes you more effective in carrying out the tasks and duties that you have to by improving your general mood.

>> Do you realize that exercising increases self-confidence and makes you able to make decisions and become a leader for yourself.

Now that we have mentioned some of the benefits of playing sports, you must be prepared to start exercising, but before that make sure you wear the right clothes and choose the right place, to exercise in , And below, I will remind you of the best sports that you can practice and will help you to maintain your health and prevent diseases.

FOOTBALL :

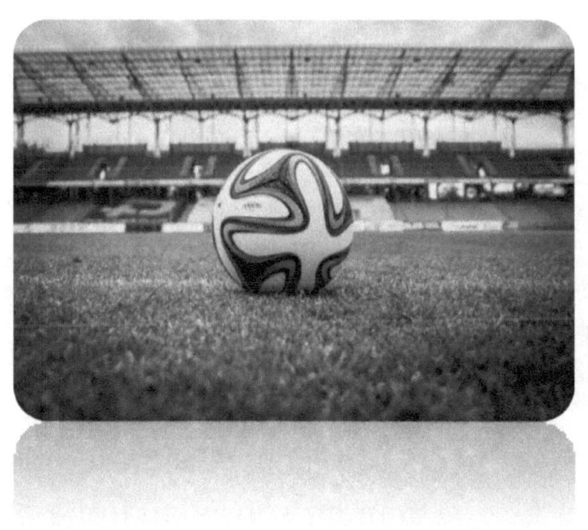

Sport is one of the most popular sports around the world, and this sport has many advantages. It combines several different functions such as running and focusing at the same time. This sport has many benefits for public health and physical and psychological health, so we advise you to practice this sport in proportion to the benefits that you will get from it in addition to improving it From your appearance and make you attractive , One of the great things about football is that it is suitable for all people and for all age groups, it is good and safe for children, as the elderly can practice from time to time to maintain their health, so we strongly recommend that you experience football as it is beautiful and lesbian at the same time.

SWIMMING : -

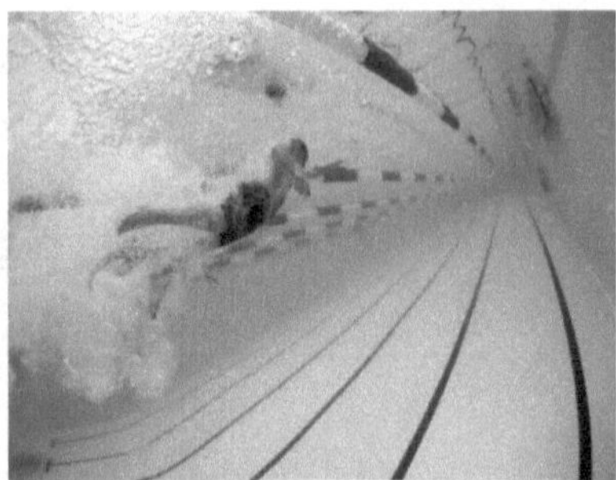

Swimming is a very beautiful sport and activities in addition to the great benefits that accrue to the health of the person exercising it, and the benefits of this sport are that it increases activity and vitality in the body in addition to improving the joints as a result of rapid wave movement , We find that most people who practice this sport enjoy high physical fitness and agility.

RUNNING:

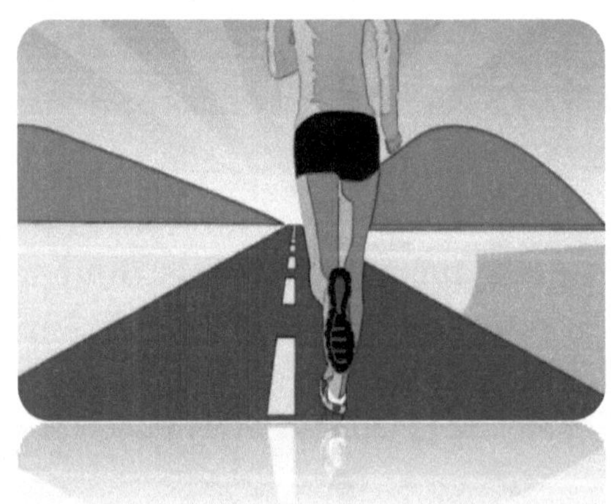

It is considered one of the most famous and known sports since ancient times, and this sport has great benefits for the personal health of individuals, besides it makes the body flexible and coordinated, It is one of the common sports and one of its advantages is that it can be invited at any time and in any place, and running helps a lot in the process of digestion in the body, so I recommend practicing this sport, especially for those who wish to reduce their weight because it gives you positive results in a short period.

WEIGHT LIFTING:

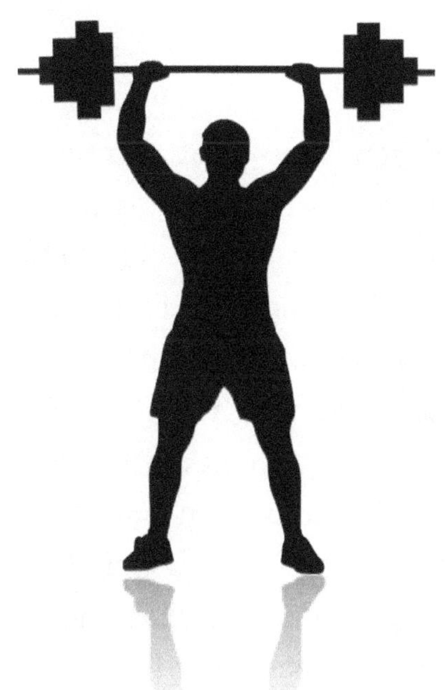

If you are one of the people who prefer to have an attractive and strong appearance and prominent and worn muscles, then you have a sport of weightlifting it is very beneficial to health in addition to its other benefits such as body coordination , But we must be cautious when exercising this sport and not to start by lifting heavy weights, as this would tear the ligaments and muscles and return you to the opposite results, so you must be careful and choose the ideal weight , It is worth noting that this sport is not suitable for children and the elderly as it leads to harm them.

PUSH-UPS:

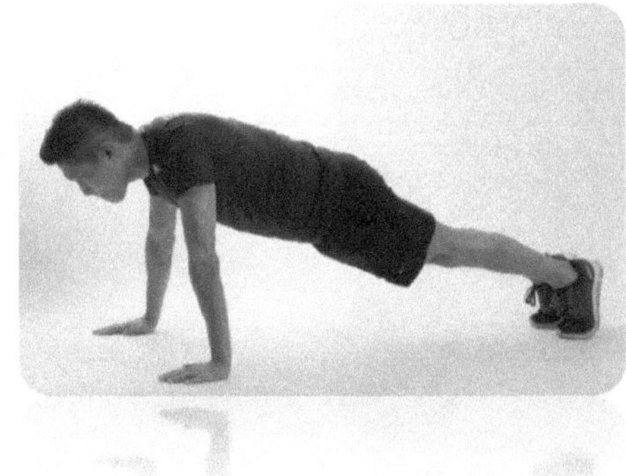

Do you need an attractive body, but you do not prefer to exercise weightlifting first? You do not have time to go to the gyms for exercise, you do not need pressure exercises to provide you with the attractive appearance and physical fitness that you need. One of the benefits of this sport is, of course, maintaining health. It works on building and enlarging muscles, especially chest muscles, and making them prominent forward , and makes you look like famous Hollywood stars and who does not want it. To this end, you just have to do push-ups.

CLIMBING STAIRS:

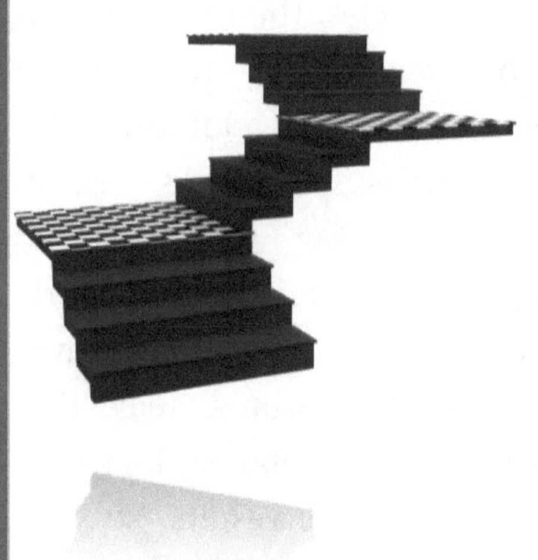

Did you know that climbing stairs is one of the recognized sports that helps you to maintain your health besides it increases the strength of determination and self-determination , So instead of going up on a lift every day, try the stairs, and so you benefit from the valuable benefits it offers you and becomes more powerful and determined.

Also, there are a lot of sports you can choose your favorite for you to practice and encourage your children to also play sports, this makes their health good and more resistant to the spreading diseases, also there are a lot of home exercises that you can practice at home and they are also useful for health and body and now to a paragraph did you know :

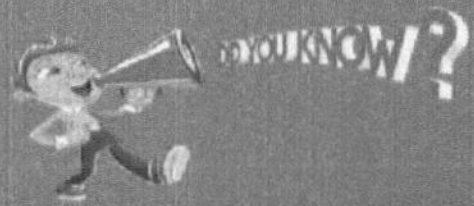

DO YOU KNOW

- Do you know that bacteria are found in abundance in the human body are found in larger quantities in the adult human body

- Do you know that the percentage of water in the brain is about 80%, so you must drink large quantities of water on a daily basis?

- Do you know that exercising early in the morning makes the body active and provides energy for the whole day

And now, dear reader, we will move on to the last chapter of our interesting book, "To prevent diseases and preserve health, but before that we go through this flower.

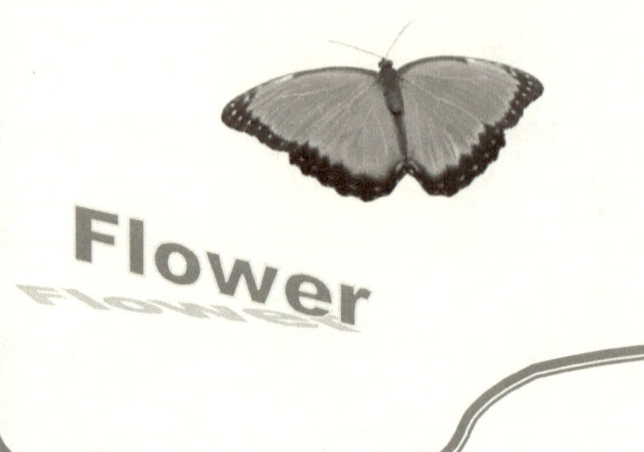

People think that feeling happy is the result of success, but success is the result of feeling happy

Marital happiness is more in the hands of the wife than in the hands of the husband

A lot of people spend time and effort avoiding problems instead of solving them

And the human scale is an estimate of the value of time

Fitness and slimming

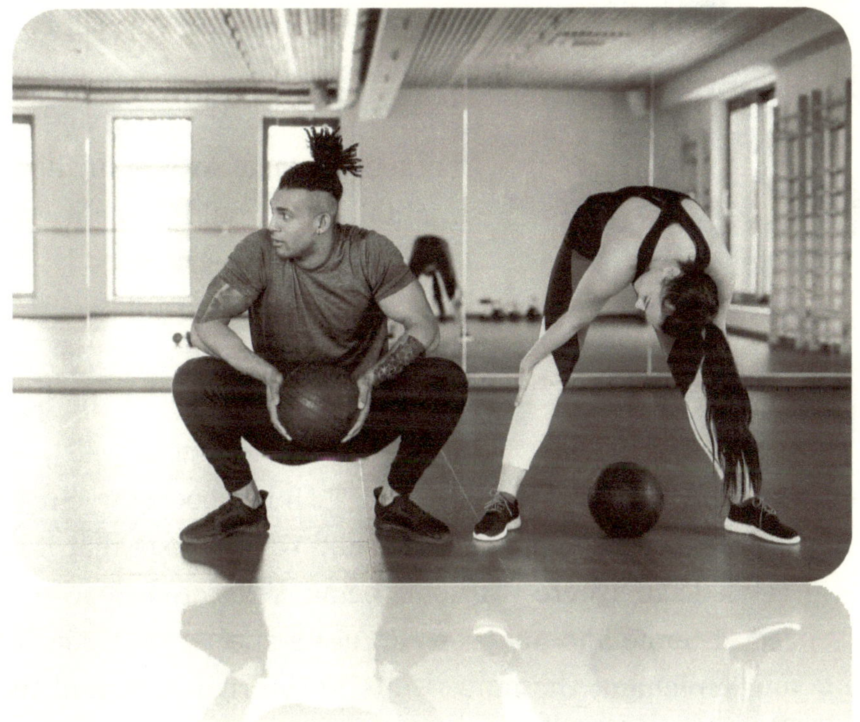

Fitness is everyone's dream, and the attractive appearance is one of the things that all people love without exception. In order to get those bodies that we see on TV, these stars pay a lot of money , But whoever told you that only stars who enjoy attractive bodies and idealism is not related to money or fame all of it is that the body interacts with the different exercises that these stars perform, which gives them that exciting body, The question is, do you want a graceful and tight body and you want an attractive and muscular body, you do not have to put you two simple exercise plan that will guarantee to you both that wonderful body in addition to the health benefits of carrying out these exercises.

YOGA:

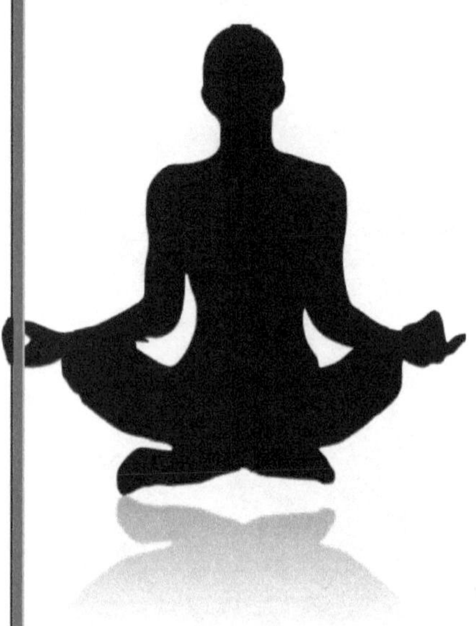

Yoga is one of the best sports for girls, because it is very simple and works on the principle of meditation and internal psychological comfort, in addition to practicing yoga with many health benefits that would benefit your health, To get a perfect body, you only have to practice this sport, as yoga contains movements that help to tighten the muscles of the body, especially the abdomen, waist, and buttocks, and this would make you a Hollywood star, So you have to practice this sport regularly and well in yoga that it can be practiced anywhere without being restricted it can be practiced at home and also you can use a special yoga coach to help you implement the movements in the right way and then you will notice a big difference.

100 PUSH-UPS DAILY:

If you want a body like the star "The rock", your climax, you should not be afraid. I will not tell you to go to the gym and start with weightlifting. The idea is very simple, which is to do 100 pressure exercises daily, and this will tighten your body and make it become the body of the stars who spend thousands of dollars for that appearance, In the beginning it will be very difficult, but never in a gradual manner such as 20 pressure exercises per day, and after that you gradually increase until your body returns to it and after only one month has passed you will find a big difference in the body of your body and you will find it has become better than the body of your friend who visits gyms constantly .

Thus, dear reader, we will have reached the end of our interesting book, which was titled " Steps for Disease Prevention and Healthy Living " and it was a very beautiful journey in which we dived into the depths of the book and the health system, and we knew the best ways to prevent diseases and preserve health , In conclusion, I want to thank you very much, dear reader, for the good follow-up and hope that we will meet in another copy of our useful book, and until then to the meeting.

The book prepared by

William Adonis

www.ingramcontent.com/pod-product-compliance
Lightning Source LLC
Chambersburg PA
CBHW051133250726
48655CB00007B/3045